Live Longer and Feel Better,

a woman's guide to guiltless HRT.

James Kolter MD

ISBN: 1-4565-6910-4
ISBN-13: 9781456569105

Acknowledgements

I would like to offer a special thanks to Dr. Winnifred Cutler for her assistance and support throughout the creation of this project. She shares my enthusiasm and concern for women's health. Similarly, Tom Quay, Esq has helped me swim through the maze of potential legalities with his insight about this project. Finally, I especially thank my wife, Pam, who has provided me with constant support in our conviction to 'do the right thing'.

❧❧

There have been studies looking into longevity over the years. One of the interesting aspects to longevity is that as you comply with the guidelines *for* longevity, you will feel better, too! That makes sense: The healthier you become, the better you feel...the positive feedback to you will reinforce your healthy lifestyle. The following points are my recommendations for women to feel better and enjoy a longer life:

1. *Maintain your endocrine (hormonal) system.* As women age, it is common for ovarian hormones and thyroid hormone to decline. The maintenance of these is a key element to the success of feeling better AND living longer.

2. *Exercise.* As little as a 30-minute daily walk has been found beneficial in virtually EVERY study, whether the end-point is longevity, heart disease or cancer incidence/mortality. You will find that as you work to carefully and moderately increase your level of exercise the better you will feel. This translates into even better outcomes! That cycle goes on and on and on...

3. *Commit to Proper Nutrition:* the Mediterranean diet and a small amount of red wine consistently have been found beneficial. The

'healthy diet' consists of fresh veggies, grains, nuts, berries, fruit and olive oil (vegetarian) plus 'white' meat up to 3 or 4 times a week (fish or chicken for example). Red wine should become a component of a healthy lifestyle for most women—up to 8 ounces a day. There appears to be a significant decrease in death rate, heart disease and even cancers if you drink wine, but in moderation and relative to your size and weight (average 5 oz glass of wine = 1 serving). These benefits do not appear to accompany beer or hard liquor.

4. *Avoid risky behavior:* This means: No Smoking (or illicit drug use), wear seat belts, do not text and drive.

I think one of the most important actions a woman can take as she approaches and enters menopause is to work with her doctor to choose the best regimen of Hormone Replacement Therapy if this is right for her. If you are lucky enough to already have reached the years far into menopause, great going and good luck to you. If not, you will need some essential knowledge to navigate smoothly through the transition called menopause.

LIVE LONGER AND FEEL BETTER,
A WOMAN'S GUIDE TO GUILTLESS HORMONE
REPLACEMENT THERAPY!

Live longer and feel better! Sounds pretty good? During the 1960's and 70's, many women heard this promise from their gynecologist. All a menopausal woman had to do was go to the doctor for an annual check-up and the doctor would give her a prescription for estrogen. There were studies showing a longer life...even better than a longer life, eternal youth! Estrogen therapy was going to keep a woman youthful in appearance and promote better health and a longer life.

It was well known that men were much more likely to die of heart attacks than women before menopause. By taking this little pill every day, a menopausal woman was told she could maintain that edge of heart health! As time went by, the medical world found even more reason to celebrate replacement doses of estrogen and progesterone. After menopause, a woman's bones tended to rapidly become brittle and prone to break: *osteoporosis.* Replacing the missing ovarian hormones helped prevent this often fatal (or at least disabling) life crisis.

Initially the prescribers did not recognize that progesterone appropriately coupled to estrogen did an even better job.

And sex became good again! After her ovaries stopped producing adequate estrogen, a woman's vaginal tissues become dry and fragile, often bleeding with even gentle sex. Once estrogen is taken, this atrophy reverses and intimacy is no longer shunned as a painful dreaded experience. The added perks of fewer wrinkles, smoother skin, better hair cinched it. 'Estrogen for all' became the mantra for many women who now had an enhanced *joie de vivre* during their menopause transition. During the last decade, hormone replacement therapy prescriptions dropped by over 50%. Doctors were actually talking women out of using these miracle hormones! And they still are. How can these wonderful benefits be denied women experiencing discomfort? What is going on with doctors?

There is an ancient fable from the Far East in which 6 blind men are asked to describe an elephant:

> The blind man who feels a leg says the elephant is like a pillar; the one who feels the tail says the elephant is like a rope; the one who feels the trunk says the elephant is like a tree branch; the one who feels the ear says the elephant is like a hand fan; the one who feels the belly says the elephant is like a wall; and the one who feels the tusk says the elephant is like a solid pipe.

So you see, each is right yet each is wrong. This is how I think of our specialists who are working to try to understand the effects of HRT. They each are "right", and have data to show it. However each is wrong for failing to explore the entirety of the dilemma. The cardiologist who studies a group of menopausal women who have previously had a heart attack do so because this group of women is fertile soil for finding results quickly. If you fit into that category of patient then the study is good for you. However, don't let this group's data be extrapolated to your case if you do not fit into that study population. Their results may not apply to you. <u>Always ask of a study</u>: *Whom* did they study and under *what circumstances*? Otherwise, the doctor is only feeling the elephant's tail!

The same goes for the discovery of breast cancer. Do not be confused and think a study proves HRT causes more cancers just because they happen to find more cancer. If HRT creates a substantial increase in the number of new breast cancers, logic would say one should find a proportional increase in breast cancer mortality in HRT users. Actually, the opposite is true! Feeling the elephant's ears?

When the medical profession started to think that smoking cigarettes could be harmful, the initial studies were circumstantial evidence to be sure, but consistent. Every study, in every way, found a link between smoking and serious illness and *death*. Then

3

confirmational studies nailed the coffin shut. Cigarette smoking kills! We do not see these kinds of data accumulated for HRT. In short, do not feel guilty or afraid you are sacrificing your longevity (health) just to feel a little (or a lot) better by taking HRT. A good HRT regimen can increase your longevity.

So what motivates doctors to do some of the things they do? Time is money. This sounds harsh, I know. However, I have worked in a busy practice for many years. I find that it takes a lot more time to explain HRT (pros, cons, is it right for me?) than to acquiesce to the supposition that it is bad overall. Easier, and more profitable to just 'move on to the next patient"! Many years ago I once worked with a doctor known to chant to the nurses, "Keep up the flow, I'll bring in the dough!"

Another thing is *fear*! Let me say that again: FEAR! Doctors are <u>afraid</u> of lawsuits, and patients have become <u>afraid </u>of taking estrogen therapy. Lawsuits? In our litigious society, lawsuits are often won or lost on emotion and not truth or knowledge. There is a huge dis-incentive created by the media hype, combined with litigation risk, preventing practitioners from looking objectively at HRT.

As a physician, I can understand the forces that drive us to think that HRT can be harmful (a 'convenient truth'?). A woman with breast cancer might win a lawsuit even though there is no direct evidence that estrogen actually caused her cancer. A physician is confronted with patients who hear from our mass media that HRT is harmful. Should the practitioner take the extra time to educate the woman about HRT only to be sued should she develop an unrelated breast cancer many years later?

After age 40, at least 5 out of every 100 women will develop breast cancer no matter what they do regarding HRT. Will I have to defend my prescriptions in court (so not only do I spend more time during the visit, but may lose days of productivity while defending myself in court)? *I have never heard of a lawsuit where a physician is accused of NOT prescribing HRT!* So what if the patient develops premature osteoporosis and finds herself in a wheelchair...no lawsuit. Or experiences painful intercourse...no lawsuit. Or develops coronary artery disease...no lawsuit. You get the picture?

So what fed the women's fear? Doctors and the Media!

The Women's Health Initiative study, as publicized, was touted as designed to help answer the questions that often plagued the practitioner. *Just how good or bad is hormone therapy?* They tested estrogen in women who had no uterus and they tested estrogen with a progestin in women who had a uterus. Unfortunately, these 2 studies, which are often cited any time anyone wants to trumpet the evils of hormone therapy, were specifically targeted to older postmenopausal women who already had evidence of arteriosclerosis, obesity, and other diseases. And it never accomplished its goals of showing benefits scientifically. Practically, however, it had such an impact that one would think it defined the pros and cons with precision.

On July 17, 2002, the Journal of the American Medical Association published the "Risks and Benefits of Estrogen Plus Progestin in Healthy Postmenopausal Women". Unfortunately, on July 15 and 16, 2002, most major news organizations ran stories decrying the harm of hormone replacement in menopausal women citing the soon-to-be-published FACTS. These *news* stories often ended with a warning to call your doctor if you are prescribed hormones for menopausal symptoms since they may be harmful! Anytime breaking medical news is released to the media before it is published, there should be caution in the wind. In this case, most gynecologists' offices were barraged with telephone calls by frightened (or at least curious) patients even before the study had been published.

So, let's look at this landmark research project. The researchers used only one estrogen preparation: conjugated horse estrogens either with a progestin (Prempro)or without progesterone (Premarin). The women all used only oral therapy. Most of the subjects were older and more than 10 years past the onset of menopause. They were largely asymptomatic yet had more underlying medical problems than younger women. The researchers concluded that the risks of taking the estrogen-progestin combination drug they used were so great that one of the studies had to be terminated prematurely. The risks from heart attacks and breast cancer were too great! Yet, according to the National Institutes of Health News published Feb. 15, 2010, when these same data were reevaluated by a more standard statistical analysis:

> "...the increased risk of heart disease was *not statistically significant*....and
> Women who started combination hormone therapy less than 10 years after menopause remained at increased risk of heart disease on average for about six years, after which those in the *treatment group appeared to have a lower risk of heart disease* compared to similar women who were not on combination hormone therapy. In the HERS study, the initially increased risk on combination hormone therapy changed toward lower risk of heart disease after about three years." (NIH News 2/15/10)

It seems that the risk for deep vein thrombosis (blood clots in leg veins) was the only adverse outcome with a statistically significant result. There was no increase death rate for hormone users, and in fact, during the last year of the study, almost a 20 % lower mortality for those on hormones than those on placebo. Interestingly, heart attacks were also about 20 % less in HRT users for the last year of data collection. Beware of any study's commentary in which the results are 'not statistically significant' but states: 'trends suggest' a result! This discourse displays observer bias and is not true science! Worse yet, it is misleading.

So what does one need to know to decide on the merits of hormone replacement? When I treat a woman in my practice, I try to follow the basics of good clinical medicine. If there is a treatment that solves most or all of the complaints, that one treatment is usually the best. Don't use 2 or 3 medicines if one will do!

What are the complaints? Do they present a problem with your daily living experiences? Do they pose a risk for the future health of your body? Do you have a family history of cardiac disease or osteoporosis that may pose a serious risk to your life or of permanent disability in later life? In short, is there a problem? Hot flashes and night sweats can lead to sleep disturbances and even symptoms of depression that can seriously affect a day's activities or performance at work.

As many as 15% of women enter and finish the menopausal changes with little or no significant symptoms. There is little reason to pursue a treatment for a condition with no symptoms. However, the majority of women will have significant problems during the change into menopause. So let's list these:

- Hot-flashes and night-sweats
- Mood swings,
- Insomnia
- Vaginal dryness (vaginal pain, especially if sexually active),
- Frequent urinary tract infections
- Diminished Bone density leading to frailty and even broken bones!

Can one diagnosis answer to all these complaints? Yes: MENOPAUSE, the age-related loss of Estrogen and Progesterone. Is there one treatment that can address all these symptoms? Again, YES. Correct the hormone deficiency.

It has always seemed odd to me that some physicians consider correcting ovarian hormone deficiency such a bad thing to recommend. It is universally recommended for women with premature menopause. Those women less than 40 years of age who enter menopause either naturally or due to surgical castration have always been strongly encouraged to correct the hormone deficiency to preserve their health. Many studies confirmed that for these women overall longevity is improved, and mortality is reduced, by replacing these female hormones. The average life expectancy in the year 1900 was approximately 50 years of age. Currently, in the United

States, the average woman's life expectancy is almost 80 years of age. Menopause, on the average, begins around 51 years of age. This is a relative new condition for women. A menopausal woman today has many more years of productive longevity than ever before. Maintaining an adequate level of female hormones should be promoted as readily as providing thyroid hormone, calcium, potassium, or any component of the human body that is deficient.

So, how much is adequate?

It depends on the woman. Not all women have signs or symptoms of hormone deficiency as they pass into and through menopause. What is good for one woman may be too much or too little for another. Using salivary levels of hormones has been studied and found to be ineffective in helping prescribe these hormones judiciously. Too much of a dose will create symptoms similar to early pregnancy: bloating, fluid retention, breast soreness, etc. Too little fails to help relieve the troubling symptoms. Sometimes a balance has to be reached with a little bit of menopause symptoms with a little of hormonal symptoms: you may feel less vaginal dryness and sleep better, but you may have some breast soreness that evaporates within a few months. In the end, most women find a dose level and frequency that satisfies most symptoms and is free of side effects.

Are all progestins and estrogens the same?

NO! There are 3 main forms of estrogen circulating in fertile women's bloodstream: estrone, estradiol, and estriol. Estrone is generally thought of as storage form of estrogen because estradiol and estrone convert back and forth into each other. Estradiol is the estrogen form that is active in most of the tissues of the body. It is synthesized by the ovaries but also by fatty tissue throughout the body. Estriol is a metabolic end product. Historically, the most widely prescribed for many years, conjugated equine estrogens obtained from urine extracts of pregnant mares has been used to relieve women's menopausal symptoms. They contain 17 different metabolites including estrone, estradiol and other substances. It may sound a bit peculiar at first to use horse estrogens for human women, but remember during the centuries of modern medicine, both plants and animals provided the resource for most medicines used to treat a wide range of maladies. For example, it is relatively recent that human insulin has been used for diabetics. During my years of training, we were prescribing pig insulin! One more word of caution, please do not equate a plant source with 'natural'. We humans are much more akin to pigs or horses than we are to any plant! The concept that a plant source = 'natural and safe' is *misguided*. I believe the over-the-counter-medicine marketing experts are trying to capture a multibillion-dollar market share based on this rather outrageous concept. For many centuries, plants have provided a source for poisons as well as medicines! Thankfully, just as *human* insulin is now commonly prescribed, so too is *human* estrogen (estradiol) and progesterone.

❧❧

Various conditions are often discussed when HRT is considered for menopausal women. Let's take a look:

CANCER!

Breast Cancer "SCARE" Tactic #1—*Don't use HRT because it will give you breast cancer, breast cells are stimulated by estrogen.*

Puberty is a time when a girl's hormones begin to rise and breast buds develop into full-blown breast tissue. It is quite understandable to assume that stimulating the breast tissue with hormones in menopause will stimulate the cancer cells as well. I have heard this at conferences full of medical doctors who treat breast cancer patients. It is not just the lay audience that is being beguiled by fear. In the case of the physicians, there is an undertow of fear of litigation for wrongly prescribing a medication. Physicians sometimes have the difficult challenge of doing what is best for the patient balanced with the lowest risk of litigation. I have attended medical conferences given by doctors for doctors in which the point driven home is we must do everything possible to avoid breast cancer even if it means your life will suffer the consequences! If a study came out showing that women who do not wear seat belts have less chance of getting breast cancer, but much greater chance of dying, they would support doing away with seat belts!! We must not lose sight of the BIG PIC-TURE: 'What is going to help me LIVE LONGER and healthier', not necessarily 'what is going to keep me from finding breast cancer?'!

Physicians should not ignore, but need to navigate, the real findings; pregnancy and breast-feeding in your youth with sky-high level of estrogen and progesterone may diminish your risk of breast cancer. One of the highest risks for breast cancer is plainly age. As a woman ages and her intrinsic estrogen levels fall, her breast cancer rate rises. Let's see how fearful (and confusing) it can be! Suppose I said to you, "Breast cancer is found at least 15% more in women who use HRT than those who don't". Then I say to you, "You are less likely to die from breast cancer if you use HRT". Well both statements *appear* true and can easily be substantiated by good medical studies. These are two different parts of our proverbial elephant.

In the practice of medicine, there can be tunnel vision just as in other fields. In studies in which investigators FIND more breast cancer, the women get more mammograms and are more likely to have breast exams (either by a doctor or a breast self-exam). Furthermore, if you study breast cancer cells in a lab, you will learn that there is a substantial lag of many years between the initiation of cancer in a cell and the diagnosis of breast cancer. Most experts will say at least 5 years will pass between **oncogenesis** of breast cancer and **diagnosis** of breast cancer. In a study of 3-5 years duration, where hormones are

14

started as the study begins, virtually every one of the women in whom breast cancer is found during the ensuing 3-5 years had the cancer in her breast before the study (and the taking of hormones) began. This means that the 15% increase in diagnosis of breast cancer is *acceleration and discovery* and *not causation* in the HRT patients!

And now, there is a growing body of evidence that approximately 30 % of breast cancers will be defeated by the body's own innate defense mechanisms, especially if we doctors do not harm your body's natural healing mechanisms with harsh therapies and stresses. The BIG SCARE from the Women's Health Initiative study was published in 2002 resulting in a huge decline in HRT over the ensuing years. In 2001, there were over 60 million prescriptions for Premarin filled by women for menopausal symptoms in the U.S. This number dropped to less than 20 million by 2005. It appears that there was a surge of "studies' looking for a link between HRT and breast cancer following the WHI.

Unfortunately (tragically) for many women, it sometimes seems that the 'publish or perish' dictum wins out over 'do the right thing'. In other words, the career enhancement of the scholar by 'publishing' wins out over the best health information for women. Data "mining" can be an intellectually dishonest way to make a point of view look like it is substantiated by statistics. For instance, did you know it was a risk factor for breast cancer for a woman to use an electric blanket? Breast cancer and electric blanket use had an association but only if the blanket user was African-American and used electric blankets for 10 years. Wait...that was not adequate to show an effect so the data were further filtered... only if those using it for more than 6 months/yr were EXCLUDED from analysis. Aha! But wait, that still did not work. How about if EVER-used vs. NEVER-used were studied: still no increase. The researchers then looked further until they found (+) results only if *currently* using HRT and used it *more than 5 yrs* but not *more than 10 yrs!!!* Sad to think someone actually went through the mental gymnastics to find some/any association.

So the real question is not what qualifies as a risk for <u>finding</u> breast cancer, but what makes for an <u>early death</u> due to breast cancer. HRT is not on *that* list!

∺∝

There are over 2 ½ million breast cancer survivors alive today and the vast majority free of signs or symptoms of persist cancer. What can they do as they live full and productive lives far beyond the onset of menopause? Are they to be condemned to the ravages of a major hormone deficiency and to endure the accelerated aging and breakdown of their bodies? Or do they have to spend extra energy and expense using 4 or 5 therapies to ameliorate their symptoms? Let's use Fosamax for the bones, Lipitor for the cholesterol metabolism, lubricating jelly for the atrophic vaginitis, fans for the hot flashes, (or a change of clothes for the times the sweats and flashes occur at work) and a wagon full of various skin and hair remedies for the cosmetic changes. Where is a cost effective approach when you want it? How about the side effects and toxicity?

Well, I reiterate: FEEL BETTER AND LIVER LONGER! Women *can* have both! Many physicians are reluctant to prescribe HRT to survivors of breast cancer for several reasons. Many think they would cause harm by promoting a hormonally sensitive tumor. Is this going to result in an increased risk of dying from breast cancer? The studies suggest the opposite.

From 1993 to present, there have been many studies published which convincingly show that women prescribed HRT after having been treated for breast cancer may not be harmed by the HRT. For more specific information and a huge eye-opening experience, please take a journey to the Internet. *Breastcancerchoices.org* displays a list of 26 studies demonstrating the safety and, in many cases, an improvement in survival in breast cancer patients who use HRT. Furthermore, before we had tamoxifen as a treatment for women with breast cancer, a synthetic estrogen called Diethylstilbestrol (DES) was considered the hormonal treatment of choice for menopausal women with breast cancer. But the

DES patients had more side effects or treatment toxicities, therefore tamoxifen was recommended and became the standard treatment.

I emphasize: this *estrogen used as a TREATMENT* for breast cancer was equally effective as tamoxifen. Now fast forward to August of 2009. A study was conducted in which a relatively "low dose" estradiol (6 mg) was found as favorable as high dose (30 mg) estradiol in treating women who had recurrence of their breast cancer despite their standard aromatase inhibitor therapy. The authors concluded that the lower dose of estrogen was preferable since the 28% favorable response rate was similar in both groups but the high dose regimen had more side effects! This ("low") dose of 6 mg is much higher than the ½ to 2 mg most commonly used to treat menopausal symptoms.

At a 2007 NIH conference, Dr. Robert Hoover, Director of Statistics at the National Cancer Institute, concluded: "We have reasonable evidence that cumulative lifetime exposure to estrogen is not a risk factor for breast cancer..."

ॐॐ

And if you do not currently have breast cancer, and you have not had a blood clot in your leg veins (DVT), a recent heart attack or stroke, or active liver disease, you can certainly consider trying HRT! But first, answer a few of these questions for yourself before you approach your healthcare provider.

- Should progesterone ALWAYS be added half the time as in a young woman's 4-week cycle?
- How does progesterone affect breast and brain tissue?
- Do you take the hormones daily or in a sequential fashion?
- Do you take the hormones orally, or would you have a different result from absorption through the skin or mucus membranes?

These questions are addressed in a wonderful book by Winnifred Cutler, Ph.D. titled: *Hormones and Your Health: The Smart Woman's Guide to Hormonal and Alternative Therapies for Menopause.* I strongly suggest anyone interested in these particular issues of HRT read her book to get an excellent perspective of this aspect of hormone replacement. It is available at www.athenainstitute.com.

*ಎ*ಎ
Uterine cancer

Cancer of the uterus can describe more than one disease. The uterus is comprised of the corpus (body), and cervix. The uterus is hollow and the lining of the inside is known as endometrium. For a fertile woman, it is the endometrium that grows during the proliferative (growth) phase and develops a secretory (secreting) phase of her menstrual cycle after ovulation under the additional influence of progesterone. The lining then sheds at the time of the menstrual period as blood vessels that had supplied the tissue with nourishment break in response to the monthly withdrawal of estrogen and progesterone. As you might suspect, its initiation is commonly hormone dependent. Cancer of the lining of the uterus is called endometrial cancer. It is this kind of cancer that could be of special concern to a menopausal woman. Historically, when estrogen was first used to treat women in menopause, the doctors found a disturbingly high incidence of endometrial cancer. They had made the mistake of treating replacement hormones with only estrogen rather than mimicking nature with both estrogen and progesterone.

It did not take very long for researchers to discover the mistake and correct it. Progesterone transforms endometrial tissue from proliferative to secretory and if prescribed in adequate ways actually lowers the risk of endometrial cancer compared to postmenopausal women taking no hormones. In other words, it is protective. Women who develop endometrial cancer usually have had a prolonged exposure to estrogen with no stabilizing effect of progesterone. This we call unopposed estrogen and is to be avoided.

In the perimenopause and certainly after menopause, when ovaries are depleted of the tissue that manufactures progesterone a dramatic decline in this beneficial hormone can be measured. Often, long before she experiences any age related decline in estrogen a perimenopausal woman is experiencing dramatic plunging of her progesterone level. This imbalance can cause excessive bleeding and is discussed in detail in Dr. Cutler's book on hormones that I recommended. Even in the post-menopausal time, women always have some estrogen because the hormone is made in multiple tissues throughout the body! Besides the ovary, the adrenal glands and even fat tissue can make estrogen. That is why we find that obese women are at higher risk for endometrial cancer, especially in menopause after her body stops making progesterone and her endometrium is continuously exposed to unopposed estrogen.

Cancer of the cervix is the other common cancer of the uterus. Related to the virus, HPV, it is outside of the scope of this book. It is not hormone dependent.

ॐ∾ॐ
Colon cancer

Colon cancer is a life-threatening kind of cancer. Even though men are affected more often than women, there is a substantial representation among women. Just fewer than 27,000 women died from colon cancer in 2005. That same year 40,000 died of breast cancer.

It is fairly clear to me that not only does HRT reduce the chances of both colon cancer and the precancerous adenoma by nearly a third, HRT also reduces colon cancer mortality! Feel better and live longer! There is speculation about why this statistic has preserved through many years and studies. The most likely explanation has to do with estrogen receptors and possible gene silencing in the molecular origination of cancerous cells. For example, the genes for estrogen receptors may play a role in the activation or inactivation of the tumor suppressor genes, thus possibly suppressing the growth of tumor cells.

୨୦୬

Ovarian cancer

Ovarian cancer is quite rare accounting for 15,000 deaths per year, a figure that is maybe _5_% that of the deaths attributed to heart disease. There has been some controversy raised about HRT and this kind of cancer in the last few years. However, the facts suggest that HRT users should not fear ovarian cancer. For instance, one of the most effective measures women can take to protect themselves from ovarian cancer is to use oral contraceptives during the reproductive years. The longer a woman uses oral contraception the greater her protection. Consider this scare tactic; the statistics that were found in the million woman study from UK (data mining?) suggest that there is an increase in ovarian cancer of 1 in over 3000 hormone-using women…but only if the woman is a current hormone user and has been using it for at least five years. A past user of HRT had the same risk as if she never had used HRT! So if a 65-year old woman has used HRT for 10 years then stops, any ovarian cancer will just go away? Smells fishy here. By 2010, it had been shown that hormone users were no more likely than non-hormone users to suffer this very rare disease. Feel better AND live longer? I say, go forward and don't let this interfere with your happiness.

᷍᷍

Cardiovascular Disease (CVD)

The biggest killer of them all! Even though many women find the scare factor of cancer to be the greatest, in my practice, I find many more women have cancer-phobia than fear cardiovascular disease. Heart disease is the BIG KAHUNA. The real killer; and, in the past, one of the main reasons doctors loved to prescribe HRT. Add up all the cancer deaths in menopausal women and you are not even close to the number of women who die of cardiovascular disease. Every year, over 8 times the number of women who die of breast cancer die of Cardiovascular Disease!

Here is what you should *know:*
- Prior to menopause, a woman's risk of CVD is remarkably lower than that of a man of the same age.
- If a woman goes through premature menopause (before age 40), her risk for CVD rises abruptly to equal that of a man.
- Lab animals that have been studied show a protective effect of estrogen on atherosclerosis, heart disease and vascular disease.
- A woman's HDL is increased and (the bad) LDL is decreased, both of these changes being beneficial and helpful in

the prevention of coronary artery disease (CAD).

· The endothelium, or blood vessel lining, remains healthier in women who use HRT.

· Damage to the vessel lining often leads to an atherosclerotic plaque and high risk for a sudden cardiac event.

· Under the influence of HRT, when vessel wall damage occurs it heals faster making for less long term damage, and there may be overall less organ damage per incident.

The Agency for Healthcare Research and Quality (AHRQ) sponsors the development of Systematic Evidence Reviews through its evidence-based practice program. In 2002, their rigorously conducted review of almost 2000 studies concluded that the average woman's risk with current HRT use was roughly 36% less than the women with no HRT. When they looked at timing, it became apparent that the majority of the improvement comes after 10 years or more of HRT use: This suggests a 36 % reduced risk of heart disease mortality if HRT was used at least 10 years! The vast majority of observational studies and their meta-analysis show no association between HRT and stroke mortality.*

*Postmenopausal Hormone Replacement-Therapy and Cardiovascular Disease
Prepared for: Agency for Healthcare Research and QualityU.S. Department of

James Kolter MD

Health and Human Services2101 East Jefferson StreetRockville, MD 20852 *Journal of the American Medical Association* on August 20, 2002

Interestingly, even in the Women's Health Initiative (Prempro) trial, the cardiac risk was rapidly reduced after the first year compared to women taking no hormones. By the last year of the study, there was approximately a 20 % reduced cardiac risk for HRT users.

My conclusion: There may be a fairly narrow window of opportunity for you to gain excellent cardiovascular protection conferred by HRT. Starting HRT before or shortly after the menopause is established gives the best results because at the younger ages there is less chance of preexisting cardiac disease. This was demonstrated in two well-designed studies The conclusion—HRT is good for healthy women early into menopause but not cardiac protective in cases of *preexisting* disease. Since then other studies have been finding similar results: total cardiovascular system related deaths are substantially lower if HRT is begun early. After taking the HRT for several years, the benefits continue to accrue as the risks regress. There is no good reason from the cardiovascular perspective to stop HRT after an arbitrary length of time, i.e.5 years as many suggest…that is when the best outcome is beginning to happen!

One final point: women in menopause who take the right HRT will feel better! That is your clue that your regimen works for you. Feel better AND live longer. The other heart-healthy lifestyle elements like exercise and proper nutrition are much easier to accomplish in women who feel well. If you are not sleepless, do not change your pajamas through the night (and blouse through the day), and therefore less depressed and/or irritable, you will be more inclined to be physically active at both work and play. You will find less vaginal dryness/painful intercourse, less osteoporosis, and less arthritic pain and you will exercise and eat healthier. All of this contributes to further lowering of cardiac risk...the number one, NUMERO UNO, cause of mortality for women!

ᐧᐧᐧ
Deep vein thrombosis (DVT)

Deep vein thrombosis has long been heralded as one of the more significant risks of using estrogen. This is true whether the estrogen comes from the ovary, placenta, birth control pills or HRT! One action of estrogen is to help your blood coagulate. Think what happens in wound healing; how your blood needs to clot to stop the bleeding. If you develop a clot in a deep leg vein and a part breaks away from the original clot, this embolus (broken piece of clot) is taken with the flow of blood through the veins. The path ultimately leads through the heart into the pulmonary arteries and into the lung where the clot can become impacted preventing blood flow. That segment of lung no longer can oxygenate blood and may become dead or infarcted lung tissue.

The occurrence of pulmonary embolism can cause: painful respiration, shortness of breath, and, most importantly, death. This is not likely to be your problem because it is rare in menopausal women compared to younger women. The occurrence is:

- 36 per 100,000 women per year using oral contraceptive
- 50-60   per 100, 000 pregnant women per year

- 11 per 100,000 women who use HRT patients show an occurrence of about per year.

Oral estrogen roughly doubles a menopausal woman's baseline risk **from 5 to 11 per 100,000.** When hormones are taken by others routes (absorbed through the skin) instead of swallowed into the digestive system there appears to be no increased risk at all. So it makes sense to individualize the method of HRT to get the best results.

There are many other risk factors for deep venous thrombosis, such as major trauma and/or surgery, many chronic and acute medical illnesses, many inherited disorders related to blood clotting, various medicines, and even obesity. **The good news is that HRT by any route other than swallowing a pill is innocent of causing the condition.**

MEMORY PROBLEMS

Thanks to several movies, such as On Golden Pond, many of us have as idea of the progressive relentless nature of Alzheimer's disease. Most women notice a decline in their cognitive abilities as they age. This seems to worsen more quickly about 10 years after menopause.

As a woman's estrogens continue to decline, her memory worsens. There have been several studies suggesting that initiation of HRT soon after the onset of menopause is accompanied by less severe and later onset dementia. A woman must have at least 8-10 years of HRT before a demonstrable improvement shows up in the studies. However, more recent studies dealing with women in whom Alzheimer's disease has already been diagnosed show only a worsening of their cognitive abilities after starting HRT. This is no surprise and is a parallel phenomenon to the cardiac dichotomy: *preventive* studies show good results but *once the disease has begun*, there is little chance to change the ultimate course favorably. Do not lock the gate AFTER the horses have gotten out!

In the brain, as in coronary blood vessels, once the plaques and tangles that impede brain function have formed, any good preventive measure is going to be unsuccessful. MRI brain studies have demonstrated significantly more brain tissue in surgically menopausal women treated with estrogens than those in a hormone-deprived state. In other words, functional and physical evidence supports this concept of HRT preserving good mental function.

If one starts HRT after the neurological disease in underway, the sluggish blood flow (as found for cardiovascular diseases) and hyper (excess) coagulation effects of oral HRT will worsen preexisting disease. In fact, I find that almost all heart-healthy actions also serve similarly well as cognition preservers! We find the hypertensive patients have more of a chance of developing memory problems just as they have increased cardiac risk. Exercise, good diet, not smoking tobacco, and maintaining a balance of female hormones are all favorable in a prevention mode for both brain and heart.

One more word of caution about what you learn from the media, the Internet and published studies. Be curious but use good judgment! Many studies tested women long after they had entered menopause. As I have demonstrated, they are testing the WRONG WOMEN for the study to apply to YOU!!! Always ask yourself: "Is this report or study about women like me? Always check out the nature of the study before you digest the results. "Alzheimer's patients get worse taking HRT!" is a common assertion and interesting, but unrelated to the basic theme of this book: Feel Better and Live Longer. Do not allow the ravages of time to get ahead of you, and then try to catch up by taking too little, too late.

꒰∾꒱

Conclusion

So do not despair menopause! True, the human body abhors change most of the time. But I hope I have shown you how, with a little common sense, accommodating these changes with a healthy attitude about diet, exercise, and a proper endocrine support system; you *can enjoy* your life during and after menopause. You can Live Longer and Feel Better!

∞

APPENDIX

Data from the (in)famous Women's Health Initiative study published in the Journal of the American Medical Association: Risks and Benefits of Estrogen Plus Progestin in Healthy Postmenopausal Women Principal Results From the Women's Health Initiative Randomized Controlled Trial, JAMA, July 17, 2002—Vol 288, No. 3

What to look for:

No increase (actually less) mortality in women using hormones during the study period. Look at the last year of the study: LOWER mortality in the treatment group! When reanalyzed with conventional statistic methods, in the estrogen only arm of the study: 10 fewer deaths, 10 fewer heart events, and 2 fewer strokes per 10,000. In the group using both e+p: 6 fewer deaths, 4 fewer heart events and 5 more strokes per 10,000 users. (JAMA 2007: 297:1465)

In the last year of WHI study, the data show: 0.78 times the rate of heart attack (over 20 % less) and 0.84 risk of dying (16% less) in hormone users. Analysis of breast cancer revealed that while they found

24% more breast cancer in the E + P group, there were actually 20 % fewer breast cancers found in the E alone group. (Stefanik.JAMA.2006:295:1647.)

> The HERS study: Hulley, S., Grady, D., Bush T., Furberg, C., Herrington, D., Riggs, B. and Vittinghoff, E. (1998) Randomized trial of estrogen plus progestin for secondary prevention of coronary heart disease in postmenopausal women. J. Am. Med. Assoc., 280, 605–613.

HERS involved 2,763 postmenopausal women, average age 67, who were treated for approximately 4 years with preexisting heart disease. Healthy women were purposely excluded from the study population. Not surprisingly, there was no significant benefit from using hormone replacement in these women.

North American Menopause Society 2010 Position Statement

The potential absolute risks published thus far for use of HT are low, particularly for the WHI ET trial, which provided evidence of considerable safety for 0.626 mg/day of oral CE. The risks in the WHI EPT trial were rare by the criteria of the Council for International Organizations of Medical Sciences, except for stroke, which was above the rare category. For women younger than age 50 or those at the low risk of CHD, stroke, osteoporosis, breast cancer, or colon cancer, the absolute risk or benefit from ET or EPT is likely to be even smaller than that demonstrated in the WHI, although the relative risk at different ages may be similar. There is a growing body of evidence that each type of estrogen and progestogen, route of administration, and timing of therapy has distinct beneficial and adverse effects. Further research remains essential.

American College of Obstetrics and Gynecology:

It is also concluded that evidence was insufficient to recommend for or against use of estrogen therapy alone for prevention of chronic conditions in postmenopausal women who have had a hysterectomy but is evaluating more recent evidence. The use of HT for specific indications, for example, treatment of menopausal symptoms or treatment of osteoporosis, will require balancing the known benefits of HTin treating these conditions with the known or potential risks of HT, as well as balancing the benefits and risks of alternatives to HT. Clearly, healthy symptomatic women who choose to use the most effective treatment for menopausal symptoms, that is, HT, should not be denied this option based on available data regarding health risks. Indeed,

based on the noted recent decision analysis (that balances benefits and risks), women using HT for several years to treat symptoms may have an improvement in quality-adjusted life expectancy.

In their monograph, Continuing Care for Women With Breast Cancer, Clinical Updates in Women's Health Care, Vol IX, No. 2, April 2010, the ACOG acknowledges that several small studies have found that women who have survived their treatment for breast cancer do not appear to have bad outcomes if they use HRT. Indeed, the studies find *breast cancer mortality* to be 5/1000 among HRT users vs 15/1000 in nonusers. *Total mortality* was also significantly lowered by one half in users of HRT vs nonusers! They concluded that data on safety of HT after breast cancer in inconclusive, and it is not known if estrogen will affect recurrence.

BREAST CANCER
RISK FACTORS;

From Cutler, WB (2009): Hormones and Your Health. John Wiley &Sons, 2009:

Behaviors the influence breast cancer:

Women 50-70years old	Breast cancer cases/10,000
Never used	45
>5 yrs HRT	47
>10 yrs HRT	51
>15 yrs HRT	57
Menopause after age 60	59
Alcohol (2 drinks/d)	72
No daily exercise	72
Weight gain (>20kg)	90

MORE RISK FACTORS
(courtesy of DATA MINING?)

From Skeptical Inquirer V.34 issue 3. P.51. The factors listed below were all reported in medical literature even though most are quite weak or not replicated in other studies. Please note the very REAL risk for lung cancer and smoking at the bottom of the list.

Risk factor	*Relative Risk breast cancer*
Conjugated equine estrogen	0.77
Fish intake	1.14
Prempro (WHI)	1.24
French fries(1 serving/wk)	1.27
Grapefruit intake	1.30
Night shift work	1.51
Flight attendant(Finnish)	1.87
Dutch famine	2.01
Antibiotic use	2.07
Left handedness(premenopausal)	2.41
Flight attendant (Icelandic)	4.10
Electric blanket use	4.90
Tobacco smoking and lung cancer	26.07

HIGHLY RECOMMENDED

* www.Athenainstitute.com

* www.Breastcancerchoices.org

*http://www.newsroom.heart.org/index.
php?s=43&item=392

* *Cutler, WB: Hormones and Your Health: The Smart Woman's Guide to Hormonal and Alternative Therapies for Menopause. Copyright © 2009 John Wiley & Sons, Inc.*